THE NEW ANCIENT DIET

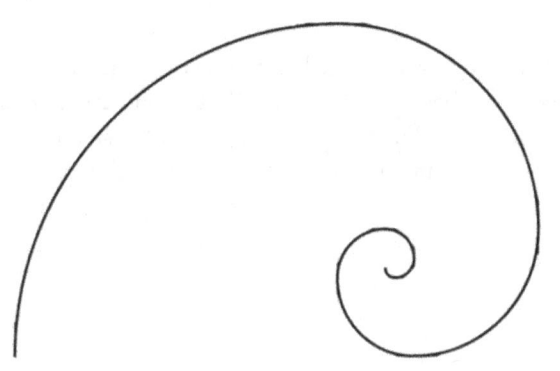

PATRICK D. ESPY, MS, RPh

The golden ratio spiral depicted on the cover and throughout this book is an ancient mathematical expression of the perfection of nature. It is used in The NEW Ancient Diet to represent the statuesque beauty of the human body that is innate to all of us.

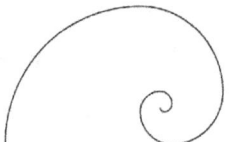

ISBN: 1500737321
ISBN-13: 9781500737320

Library of Congress Control Number: 2014913936
CreateSpace Independent Publishing Platform
North Charleston, South Carolina

To my sunshine,
Elle and Ivan

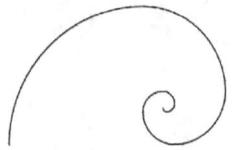

TABLE OF CONTENTS

INTRODUCTION

The significant problems we have cannot be solved at the same level of thinking with which we created them.
— Albert Einstein

Even though Einstein was a man of science, his wisdom rings true in all aspects of our lives and reaches us now in a modern world filled with modern problems. Our generation faces problems like the health care crisis, our dependency on oil and a struggling economy and we understand that in order to solve these problems, we need to approach them with a fresh mind.

I propose the question, "Why are we not doing the same with the obesity epidemic?" The way Americans consume food has changed dramatically over just the last fifty years, and not enough of us have stopped to consider that. We now get many of our meals from within our cars at fast-food restaurants, or we sit on our couches and eat them inactively. The world has changed around us, and we Americans have not adjusted our thinking along with it.

In case you haven't heard, according to The National Institutes of Health, over two-thirds (68.8 percent) of Americans age twenty or over are considered to be overweight or obese.

So, yes, just to be clear, *this is an epidemic.*

It is going to take a very meaningful and massive shift of thinking for our country to combat this, because so many people either don't know how to lose weight or have nothing but misconceptions and misinformation on the subject.

An example of this misinformation began in the 1990s, when many believed that the model example of a great diet was to eat six smaller meals a day to stoke the metabolic fire. This system is still utilized by many. While this method can be helpful for people who use dramatic supplements and have extreme bodybuilding goals, the reality is that others following this program do so at their own detriment.

I'm trying to let the world know that we need to completely overhaul our thinking when it comes to how we diet and exercise to lose body fat. This topic has long been a passionate project for me; this has been a book thirty years in the making. That's how long I've had a passion for learning everything I could about fitness.

When I was just a boy at age eleven, I begged my parents to get me a barbell set for my room. My poor mother had to deal with her eleven-year-old who wanted to push his body weight over a delicate skeleton.

I couldn't help it. Even at eleven, the fire was there.

I had gotten the idea from muscle magazines my father and uncles would leave sitting around. In the mind of one eleven-year-old boy, the guys in those magazines represented everything a man was supposed to be. They must have walked the earth as gods among men if they were worthy enough to grace the covers of my father's bathroom reading. With my new weight set, I could finally get *strong* and *lean* like those guys in the magazines, and I would have it all:

@ women

@ a fantastic body

@ the strength of three men

@ women

So I wanted to be a bodybuilder. I wanted that, and I wanted it badly. I was totally hooked. I knew I didn't have the best genetic makeup or body type for bodybuilding, but that wasn't about to stop me. My passion was set.

I constantly devoured all the bro science (and actual science) I could get my hands on. Over the next several years, I read and experimented with just about everything I could in relation to bodybuilding and body composition, and after, I eventually upgraded to a real gym membership. I tried all the popular bodybuilding routines of the day: Nautilus, Weider, Arnold, etc. They all had their value, but after reading up, talking to experts, and generally observing, I realized that it wasn't going to be enough to just work out. If I was going to be great (and I was sure I was), I had to keep a smart eye on my diet as well.

This was the 1980s, and in case you weren't there, fitness and body-building were all about carbs and calories. So naturally, I ate tons of carbs and calories (I'll talk more about carbs later).

That's how my quest to find the ultimate diet and exercise routine for getting the quickest results started: a man who basically carb loaded.

Speed up to 2012: I've tried every single diet and exercise program out there. Along the way, I developed a strong science background, becoming a pharmacist and even earning a master's degree in exercise physiology (one of my proudest personal accomplishments). I also never stopped practicing my mantra: train hard; diet hard. But in order to continue my undertaking of finding the absolute most efficient diet and exercise methodology, I still had a lot of experimenting to do.

My method was simple and pragmatic: whatever works, keep doing it. And of course, whatever doesn't work went back on the shelf. I evaluated every diet and exercise theory on three levels:

1.   Does it work on a practical level?

2.   Are there reputable studies showing that it works?

3.   Does it make good sense biologically and based on our history as a species?

So if I heard of a new training method or diet making its rounds, then I would always evaluate it based on practicality, science, and history. Then I'd incorporate anything that passed through those three gates and discard the rest. I loved reading the science and bro science behind fitness and would take it all through my three filters to see if it was good enough to apply to my own training and diet.

All that I did led me down a constant road of self-improvement, and the results were palpable. I refined my method, constantly continued my progress, and I looked great. Heck, I even felt great.

Everything was going fantastic with my training and dieting for a long time. But the day finally came when I hit a wall.

As I entered my fourth decade of life and what some would call middle age, I began to notice that my workouts were becoming less effective than they once were. My diet hadn't changed much, nor did my training, but *something* had changed. I wasn't able to keep up the gains that I was used to. My body fat was slowly creeping up, my workouts were getting progressively less aggressive, and I was becoming honestly depressed because of it.

My physical fitness had taken a blow.

My emotional state was poor.

Even my mental health seemed diminished; it was harder and harder to keep hold of my thoughts, and it was taking me longer than ever to piece things together.

I didn't understand at all what had changed. My twenties and thirties had been fantastic, but now, my fitness seemed to be in an unstoppable decline. Nothing I tried was working, and it was beginning to look like a major problem with no solution.

Was I just getting old? Was it something worse?

I confess I had entered something of a midlife crisis, and I needed answers.

So I began a new quest: find out what the heck was happening to my body. This new mission began at the doctor, as quests of health often should. After describing my symptoms and loudly wondering about them to the doctor, he agreed to run some tests. When they finally came back, he informed me that they were all negative and there was nothing indicating I was anything other than a normal man of my age. He told me I was just fine and that I was suffering from *nothing more than getting older.*

Nothing more than getting older.

Than getting older.

Getting older.

Nothing.

This was obviously unacceptable. *Yes,* I was getting older, and *yes,* that changes things, but that doesn't mean I was willing to watch my health and fitness suffer for it. Fitness had been my passion for over thirty years, and letting it slowly slip away was not on my to-do list.

Doctors are fantastically important members of our society; there's no one better to go to when you're sick or hurt. But I wasn't sick or hurt.

The symptoms I had were mostly general, and all my tests came back normal.

I was beginning to learn that doctors help you with health, but that doesn't mean they can always help you with fitness.

I was still convinced that there was something wrong with me, so I decided that I had to handle the problem on my own. With the Internet at my side, I dove in. From peer-reviewed studies and fitness articles to simple bro science, I read it all. After swearing I had done more research then I ever had in college, I had a possible answer: **Insulin resistance**.

Insulin resistance in a nutshell: Insulin is a hormone that plays a key role in allowing your body to use food energy and convert it to movement and growth. Insulin resistance is a disease that occurs when insulin no longer works and your body loses its ability to effectively store and utilize calories. It often comes as a result of lazy inactivity and body fat buildup, and then leads to higher levels of inactivity and body fat. It's a disastrous downward spiral I hope to help you counter and avoid!

I felt like I had an aha moment. I wasn't 100 percent sure of this self-diagnosis, but it explained everything that was happening to me: the lowered energy levels, the increased body fat—all of it. I decided to move forward under the absolute assumption that I was living with insulin resistance.

My Plan in Two Points

Contrary to the wisdom of several smarter men, I began to treat myself. I was determined to do everything I could to combat insulin resistance. As I did my research, I slowly began working out two main points in my fitness battle plan.

First Fitness Point: Personally Modified Fasting.
At the time I knew of several peer-reviewed studies that had shown that insulin resistance can be tamed with fasting, so I began fasting twenty-one hours of every single day. I left myself a three to four hour window of time every day, during which I consumed my whole day's-worth of food and calories. This alone showed tangible effects: immediately my workouts got better and my body fat was melting away once more.

Second Fitness Point: 3-Hour Window Consumption.
In addition to only eating during a short period every day, I did one more thing: I forced myself to only eat when I had recently done a workout. I would consume all of my daily calories only after a daily workout.

For me, the second technique, *combined with the first one,* meant that I was consuming a whole day of calories after a single aggressive workout in a three- to four-hour period and then fasting again.

The scientific journals and peer-reviewed studies backed this up too: only eating after a workout also combats insulin resistance.

So, of course, these two diet manipulations passed my special evaluations too: they worked on a practical level, peer-reviewed studies supported them, and biologically, they made sense (I'll go into the science and biology later).

I had done these two things to combat insulin resistance, and all my symptoms disappeared. The self-diagnosis was complete. I was now certain that I was dealing with insulin resistance, because there I stood, feeling like I was in my twenties again. These two simple diet manipulations did more than correct the problem; they put me *back on top of my game.*

And if I'm going to be honest with you, I actually *still* have not been officially diagnosed with any kind of insulin-resistance problems. So looking back, I can't really be certain if that was the case or if I should have taken the doctor at his word and accepted that I was just getting older.

All I do know is that thinking that I had insulin resistance led me to this new method—this new *idea*—and my health has never been better.

And I still haven't gone back to that doctor, or any other, for a follow-up appointment.

Now that I've been doing this and using my method for years, everything is back to normal. And I'm thrilled to report that I haven't *really* suffered or sacrificed at all to do this. It's actually enjoyable. I still eat everything that I normally eat; I just manipulated my biological schedule.

My mind is clearer too, by far. Clearer and happier. Not only has good health directly yielded positive effects on my brain chemistry, not needing to obsess over my diet and exercise like I did has freed my mind from that stress.

Ever since I started doing this, I've felt like I flipped a switch in my body. It made me suddenly feel strong, full of energy, and mentally clearer than ever before. I know that some people think I'm crazy when I tell them about this, but, believe me, it works fantastically.

If you don't have any of the problems I did, then you've got a healthy leg up on me. But this program definitely isn't just for the insulin resistant.

If you're looking to have more energy, look leaner, feel sexier, increase cognition, and be a better you, then the core concepts of my method can help improve your life.

In fact, I fully believe these core concepts can help improve anyone and everyone's lives. If optimal fitness is your goal, then utilizing these techniques is a great way to get there—no matter who you are!

If you *are* experiencing the same issues I was, then I really do urge you to adopt my method—ASAP. Don't wait for a better you. I guarantee you will feel healthier and look leaner *almost immediately*.

As I'll show in the upcoming pages of this book, the techniques I discuss hold great value for anyone who's looking for his or her best self.

The goal of The NEW Ancient Diet is to get your body fat low to achieve your best self. I mean to *wow* levels: 9 to 21 percent body fat.

As you read on, *don't lose sight of that goal.* There are six big reasons you should get on board with The NEW Ancient Diet, and I call these The Big Six.

THE BIG SIX

1. It's easy: work out, and then eat. Also, there is very limited meal planning involved.

2. Limited hunger: once you become accustomed to it, you have almost no hunger. Compared to diets where you simply *eat less*, you'll feel quite satisfied.

3. No food choice restriction: you can eat whatever you want.

4. Fast results: you will start to notice body-composition changes and mind changes immediately.

5. Effectiveness: this diet is simply the most effective way to get from A to B. You want to lose the most body fat? The NEW Ancient Diet is ideal for you.

6. Happiness: as your metabolism improves, The NEW Ancient Diet makes you mentally *sharper,* and it leads to making you happier as well. It doesn't even feel like you are on a diet.

Part one of this book discusses insulin resistance in detail: what it is, what causes it, and how to fix it.

Part two discusses how to fine-tune your diet and training to get maximum results.

Finally, part three shows how to get the maximum motivation from your new diet and exercise lifestyle and how to reach the optimal you.

This is my passion. As you read and (hopefully) enjoy this book, try to start living what you're reading. As you incorporate this book into your day-to-day life, you'll start to see the best *you* ever come forward. You won't be disappointed with your results. Never lose sight of believing in yourself; you are worth it. This diet will help you to get reconnected with the real, brighter, happier you. Excellence is always within you.

Bring your excellence out with The NEW Ancient Diet.

PART ONE
INTRODUCING INSULIN

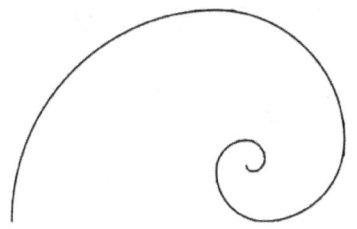

CHAPTER 1
INSULIN OVERUSE

Obese people and those desiring to lose weight should perform hard work before food. Meals should be taken after exertion and while still panting from fatigue. They should, moreover, only eat once per day and take no baths and sleep on a hard bed and walk naked as long as possible.

—Hippocrates, c. 420 BC

Hippocrates was smart. So am I. While there are some obvious differences of opinion and time that separates us, another thing we have in common is our goal to deconstruct complex problems.

Hippocrates was limited to the knowledge of his era, so I had the advantage of building on his and others' theories until they became a powerful working model of health and fitness. Once I trimmed the fat from his theories (no, I do not endorse abstaining from bathing, walking naked as long as possible, or sleeping on a hard bed), I kept only what held true value. From there, I created a new (yet very old) way to trim the fat from your life.

You see, our human bodies haven't changed in the two thousand years since he wrote that; human anatomy and biology were the same then as they are now. Thus, much of the wisdom of Hippocrates still applies to us. Taking meals after exertion and only eating once per day are the pillars that hold my method up. He may not have had the means we have to observe and study the human body, yet the truth was there.

That being said, we can't ignore the technology of nutrition science that he didn't have. So I will be applying my contemporary thoughts as well. You do not have to be "still panting from fatigue," as he recommended. I've observed that eating within about three hours is fine. Hippocrates didn't know that timing your food in this way leads to maximum insulin sensitivity, but he did observe all the good that would come of it.

Also, Hippocrates didn't mention controls on calories, carbohydrates, protein, or fat.

Well…that's where the science and nutrition knowledge of today also comes in.

INSULIN

These ideas have everything to do with a very important hormone called insulin. Insulin is a protein hormone formed and released from the pancreas that allows (*and limits*) the storage of nutrients (food) in the cells.

Basically, this makes insulin a calorie-storage hormone, as opposed to a calorie-spending hormone (like the common stress hormones adrenalin and cortisol). It's very important for a person to balance his or her internal store-versus-spend hormonal ratios to maintain optimal health and achieve a higher level of fitness.

Now, when I say that insulin regulates the storage of calories, I neglect to mention that it has a hand in the breaking down and storage of all nutrients (carbohydrate, protein, and fat), basically playing a part in the regulation of all sources of energy for your body. Many people do not understand the significant role that insulin plays in fitness and, therefore, find themselves experiencing the problems I went through.

Understanding insulin will help you use it to your advantage instead of dealing with the troubles that arise when you neglect it.

To help you understand insulin better, I'd like you to picture a lock-and-key mechanism. Insulin is the key that unlocks the door (cell opening) to allow the guest (nutrients) inside the home (into the cell). So insulin allows nutrients to enter the cell.

Some additional, important things to note about insulin:

- Much less insulin is required for fat to enter the cell at the major sites of nutrient disposal: your muscles, fat, and liver.

- Much more insulin is generally required for carbohydrate and protein to enter the cell at the major sites of nutrient disposal: your muscles, fat, and liver.

- But it's *not always* required; there is one important exception.

The major exception helps make my method work: something different happens after you work out. During a short period after you work out (about three hours, specifically), insulin is actually not required for nutrients to enter the muscle cells. As you'll see later, this is actually a very good thing. If you work smarter—not harder—you can use this to your advantage to achieve much lower levels of body fat and higher levels of fitness, health, and overall well-being.

INSULIN RESISTANCE

Everything I'm describing about the function of insulin occurs in normal, healthy human beings. Certain things like chronic overeating, eating too often, and under-exercising causes body fat to accumulate. The excess fats stored inside the body fat (pro-inflammatory belly fat, primarily) are sent around the bloodstream as metabolites (break-down products), where it accumulates in liver and muscle cells. This fat metabolite accumulation in liver and muscle cells disrupts the primary function of each: energy balance (liver) and movement or contraction (muscle).

This disruption of function is due to the fact that the fat metabolite accumulation prevents insulin from allowing transport of nutrients into the cells. This condition is called insulin resistance and is really a protection mechanism to guard against excess nutrients entering the cells, which can be toxic.

Therefore, a person with high body fat and subsequent insulin resistance produces insulin, but the receptors in muscle and liver cells (and fat cells, to a lesser degree) don't respond to insulin to allow carb, protein, and fat (to a lesser degree) metabolites to enter.

In other words (because of overeating, eating too often, under-exercising, and excess fat), the lock-and-key mechanism doesn't work properly or efficiently anymore. The metabolites of carbohydrates (aka, blood sugar or glucose), protein, and fat begin to build up in the blood because they can't enter the cells. *This results in a person's pancreas pumping out more and more insulin to do the same job.*

This extra insulin works for a while to activate the cell receptors to lower blood sugar, protein, and fat, but it continues to make your body more and more resistant to insulin.

But sometimes the additional insulin produced by the pancreas is not enough. Metabolites of carbohydrate, protein, and fat can then build up in the blood chronically; this is how insulin resistance can lead to diabetes.

Diabetes. Metabolic syndrome. Syndrome X. These are all side effects stemming from the same problem: insulin resistance due to excess body fat.

It gets worse; once a person has developed insulin resistance, the food that he or she eats is preferentially shuttled to fat cells before muscle. This is because insulin resistance occurs to the *greatest extent* in muscle cells and liver cells and lastly in fat cells. It's an unfair and brutal truth, but it can be quite a vicious circle. The more food you eat, the more food your body sends to the fat cells—and the less food that goes to the liver for energy and to the muscle for contraction.

So you get more and more body fat with less and less energy because your liver and muscles aren't being fed; your fat is.

Actually, you get a lot more body fat. Unless you find a way to undo what damage has been done.

It is very important to note that insulin resistance is the main cause of **low energy**, poor workouts, and tiredness. This is independent of age or any other disease state. Insulin resistance makes us tired, slow, and lethargic—period.

So, with insulin resistance, you gain body fat AND become more tired, and thus, the motivation and energy to do something about it become *very* hard to find.

To quote James Hetfield of the great Metallica, it's "sad but true."

Anywhere I roam in America, most adults are considered over-weight or obese, and thus, they do have a problem with insulin resistance. This means that having some degree of insulin resistance is the current normal in our society. It's an epidemic, and nothing else matters.

The normal, standard American diet (SAD) is a great example of what not to do: overeating, eating too often, under-exercising, and not planning your caloric intake around exercise. Once someone develops insulin resistance, he or she will typically experience a battery of all sorts of not-really-terrific symptoms:

- higher blood pressure

- higher cholesterol

- higher blood sugar

- lowered cognitive processes, or brain fog (literally not feeling like yourself)

- inability to lose weight

- lower testosterone

- lower sex drive

- lower energy

- depression

- premature aging

Notice that the problem we've been discussing is called "insulin resistance," not "carbohydrate resistance" or "carb intolerance." Many low-carb crusaders mistakenly believe that carbohydrates are the direct and singular cause of insulin resistance. It *is* true that carbs do contribute to the problem, but don't put the blinders on and start to think that you're looking at the full picture. Insulin is released most from eating refined carbs, but it is also released when you eat protein and other carbs as well.

Track with me on this: Insulin is like a drug or like caffeine. The less you use of it, the higher your sensitivity to it. The more you use of it, the higher your resistance to it. The reality is that anything you eat will cause your insulin to rise, thereby increasing your resistance (like increasing your tolerance). It is true that lowering carbs in your diet will help lower the total insulin created and, in turn, help with insulin resistance. However, because protein, fat, and other calories raise insulin levels too, lowering the total food/calorie intake is what truly reverses it.

Don't get me wrong; refined carbs are unhealthy for several reasons, least of which is the extra insulin spike that they cause. But restricting just the refined carbs in your diet will only help correct insulin resistance and body-fat percentage levels in a *very* limited way. The most important things for you to do are limit total food/calorie intake and adjust the timing of your meals around your exercise program.

So how does one go about fixing insulin resistance (which is to say, increase insulin sensitivity) and get body-fat percentage back down to a respectable digit? Well, brace yourself. Are you seated? You best take a seat.

1. Lower your caloric intake (e.g., eat less food).

2. Work out (e.g., exercise).

3. Time your calories after exercise (this is where my system comes in).

What I'm saying is, whether you eat chicken breasts and broccoli or Twinkies every day, total calories and caloric timing (in relation to exercise) matter most. However, remember to get enough protein (Twinkies may not be as useful here), which I will talk about later.

It's simple, right?

The details and intricacies get more complicated, of course (that's what this book is for), but the fundamental idea is that simple. Now, to burn fat, you have to burn off more calories than you eat. By necessity, the following must be true:

$$\text{calories burned} > \text{calories eaten}$$

Simply eating less calories is, unfortunately, the only tool you really have for lowering *calories eaten*, which helps you get the right side of the equation tipped in your favor. This gets you 50 percent of the recipe for quick, effective fat loss.

Most people probably think that exercising more must be the only tool they can use to adjust the left side of the equation. But this book is here to introduce to you a cheat. A sneaky life hack I call *"proper caloric intake timing"* helps you burn off more calories and more efficiently, even with the same amount of effort during workouts.

A lower-calorie diet is a great way to correct insulin resistance and shed fat, but this is a way to make it much, much easier.

Allow me a brief moment of fitness-nerd science talk. Remember when I mentioned that insulin isn't required immediately after you work out?

Well, that means that after a workout, the receptors on the muscle cells that allow food to enter are activated independently of insulin.

This leads to something pretty fantastic: the food you eat post-workout (within about three hours) is preferentially stored in muscle cells and used for energy instead of being stored in fat cells.

Bear with me, and I'll explain this in more detail. Food can only be used by muscle cells to create movement, so when your food goes there, it's actually doing something. Fat cells don't contribute to movement (at all); they just kind of exist. When your food goes to the fat, it just makes your fat get bigger.

But, when you eat immediately after you work out, you use the food as muscular energy first, independent of insulin. This means that you're using more calories and using those calories more efficiently than you would if you ate normally, without exercising first and needed the extra insulin to complete the process.

Don't get me wrong, insulin is very important to your health, but these things are similar in that the more your body produces insulin (or the more you "use" it), the higher your resistance will be (like alcohol or drug tolerance). And just like with alcohol, the less you use, the higher your sensitivity. So doing this and decreasing the amount of insulin your body needs/creates will increase your insulin sensitivity, thereby decreasing insulin resistance.

Here's some more good news: eating after exercising is going to decrease your insulin usage *whether or not* you're on a lower-calorie diet. And the more your body shuttles the energy from food to your muscle cells instead of to your fat cells, the better your body's metabolism and calorie burning is going to be. So is that one of the reasons why elite athletes can eat a lot and not put on fat? Believe it or not, I know the answer. YES.

Lil' bit of wisdom:

It's easy to see just how powerful this method is. The Calories Burned side the equation is affected to a much greater extent by shuttling food to active muscle versus stagnant fat, *and* you use a lot less insulin in the process. Eating after you workout gives you the best of *everything*:

- Food preferentially goes to active-muscle fuel replenishment and burning. You burn a lot more fuel (calories) and get more energy stored for the next workout, instead of stored in fat.

- You trick your body into minimum use of insulin: Thus your insulin sensitivity increases further.

- You get minimum fat storage after the workout because the food you just ate is going to active-muscle to be used for fuel and burning, instead of fat storage.

You probably already knew this on a basic, intuitive level but never really drew the thought out: letting your muscles use the calories for movement is far better than letting it go to your fat cells for storage. But it gets a little bit more complicated.

This method is all about getting your body to use the fuel you give it most efficiently, like tricking out your car to get higher performance levels. Well, if you want to push this method to get your body to burn more calories in the *absolutely* most efficient way possible, there's another piece to the puzzle: you need to eat ONLY after you work out. Not before—at all.

This means you shouldn't eat at all before you work out. To do this, fast the other hours of the day (This is assuming that you are working out only once daily, which is my recommendation. However, I will mention twice daily eating/workouts in chapters 2 and 3). This can sound really intimidating at first, but it's a simple manipulation that does bountiful wonders for your metabolism.

Like I said, most of us have some understanding of these things on a basic level, but more than that, most people already practice pieces of my method to a limited extent. After all, we don't eat *every hour* of the day. We do mini fasts daily—eight to fourteen hours—while we sleep. Breakfast literally means "break the fast." What I'm recommending is taking that walk just a few steps further. Fast just a little longer...

Twenty-one hours total, to be exact.

Then, *voila!* You get tons of physiological (and as I'll talk about later, psychological) benefits.

And this, my friends, gets you the other 50 percent of the recipe for amazingly quick, effective fat loss.

In summary, to get 100 percent of the recipe for amazingly quick, effective fat loss, do two very important things:

@ Eat a *lower*-calorie diet.

@ Eat *only* after you've recently worked out.

CHAPTER 2

CLOSER

The soul of The NEW Ancient Diet is to eat only after you have recently worked out, but the twenty-one-hour fast improves your insulin sensitivity even further. And having a controlled (but doable) amount of calories helps rid your body of fat quicker than these two points alone.

Having one meal a day makes eating only after you work out a more manageable task. That being said, if it's better for you, it's still OK to apply caloric intake timing to two meals a day after exercise. This is still better than not timing your calories at all, but one properly timed meal a day is often easier to fit into your schedule and does provide the additional benefits that come with daily twenty-one hour fasting.

I'm expecting that you will quickly become a believer in this diet, but maybe you are not yet sold on this eat-for-only-three-hours-a-day-idea.

If so, then I want you to ask yourself the following question. Why don't ancient paintings and sculptures depict overweight/obese people? The answer is because there were few overweight/obese people that existed back then. Before the last 100 years, people were lean. Obesity was rare, but unfortunately, it is not now. In fact, since the beginning of our time as humans on earth, we have typically practiced a type of eating pattern that entailed "working for our food." That is, eating only after we've recently done manual labor, hunted or farmed (aka, exercise, workout). That was, by design their only option, because they had to work to eat to survive. Look at ancient cultures such as the Egyptians, the Greco-Romans and the early Europeans. They ate one large meal per day after hard work and that was typical (Q: Do you think that the Pyramids of Giza in Egypt were built by laborers on 3-6 meals per day? A: No!). And that type of eating pattern gave them many major benefits, notably: extreme leanness, strength and insulin sensitivity. Humans of today do not share any of those benefits, sadly. That is because it's only been very recently in our human history, the last 50 to 100 years, that we have moved to three meals per day without regard to exercise. So, if you want those benefits, then you need to embrace and accept how our ancestors thrived. By reconstructing the past and deconstructing the present, only then can you truly and intelligently construct your leaner, fitter future.

Are you still kind of skeptical?

That's OK. I was too, but I'll admit something to you: I'm a bit of a perfectionist. I've tried *a lot* of diets and researched *a lot* to find the ideal one. So trust me when I say this: The NEW Ancient Diet is ideal and will have nothing short of a perfectly profound effect on your body composition. And, just keep in mind that this diet was developed to help you lose the most body fat in the shortest amount of time. Given that, let me clear up some common confusion with a quick Q&A.

Isn't breakfast the most important meal of the day?

No, the timing of your first meal isn't nearly as important as it's made out to be. One of the main reasons people worry about breakfast so much is that they mistakenly believe that breakfast is good for you. Breakfast in itself isn't good for you, nor is it necessarily bad for you. It's just the arbitrary nature of it that makes it not good.

A problem could arise between breakfast and my diet because breakfast is typically eaten BEFORE exercise, and that's what we're trying to avoid. Keep in mind, I'm not bagging on breakfast; in fact, I'm a morning workout person myself, so I typically eat all my daily food before two o'clock in the afternoon. So as long as you only eat any ONE time a day, you can make it breakfast, lunch, dinner, or late night. So breakfast, lunch, and dinner are OK—you just have to work out first.

If I don't eat three to six times a day, then won't my metabolism go into starvation mode?

No, the opposite is true. In fact, studies have shown it. If you have regular, controlled, short fasts (twenty-one hours), your metabolism increases instead of slowing down. Another benefit to *not* eating three to six times a day: you'll burn more fat *preferentially* over muscle. The reality of the situation is that eating once a day isn't crazy at all. It might be crazy not to.

But all the bodybuilding and fitness magazines say that you should eat three to six small meals a day. Are they are all wrong?

Yes and no. Are you trying to bodybuild competitively? If so, then three to six meals a day may be right for you. If you have the genetics, motivation, and needles to do so, keep doing what you're doing, my friend.

The six-small-meals phenomenon began for extreme bodybuilders. Many of them (especially those using steroids) would find my meal plan difficult because their diet often requires ridiculous amounts of calories that would be difficult to consume in a single meal.

But *even if you're bodybuilding*, keep in mind that most studies suggest that, once you adjust for calories and protein, one meal per day is actually superior to multiple meals per day. This is, of course, regarding maximum body-composition gains (max fat loss and muscle retention) as the goal.

And if you are still not 100 percent convinced and still asking, "Why not eat three to six times a day?" read this one more time (slowly if you have to): *eating once a day is just better for body composition*. It's the best food timing for killing body fat. Meaning you lose much more fat when eating once per day.

Also, we are an obese nation that is culturally conditioned to eat three to six times a day. Eating three to six times a day is what the standard American diet is currently based on, and clearly that is not working.

So if you're looking to start seeing your favorite body (with no needle marks) in the mirror every day; if you're looking for an easy and effective way to shed your extra body fat; or if you're just looking to be the best you, then, yes, I'm saying that three to six meals a day is wrong for you. And just because three to six *does* work for some competitive body builders, this myth has picked up way too much steam, and many have started to believe that it's right for all body types with different body-composition goals. Your body will thank you when you change things up and start feeding it the way it is *meant to be fed*.

Won't I be hungry all day long?

No, because you *are still* eating a full day of calories. At first you will notice some hunger as the day pushes closer to mealtime, but once your body has adjusted its *hunger clock*, it won't expect food more than once a day. Then you won't be feeling hungry until you're ready to eat. Like any diet, you will feel some hunger when you cut your calorie intake below the amount of calories your body burns to help shed fat. That's to be expected. There's no way to avoid that when your body is used to much higher calories than it's getting. But if you're expecting that this diet will lead to a constant nagging hunger because you're going for longer periods without eating, then put your worries to rest. Once this method is habit, you'll experience only normal hunger.

This diet sounds difficult. Isn't it hard to do?

Is the Pope Protestant? Nope.

Your brain is a more powerful tool than you could ever imagine; you can do anything if you put your mind to it.

Again, getting in the rhythm of it is the only difficult part. It requires breaking comfortable daily habits and routines. Once you've established my method as the replacement routine, it literally becomes enjoyable for many reasons. Some of those reasons are:

- © mentally clearer thoughts throughout the day (insulin resistance is gone)

- © one meal per day is very satiating/satisfying

- © no more being obsessed with meal planning and eating every three hours

CHAPTER 3
STARTING LINE

Consciously timing your food intake for after you work out is what I'm advocating here. I know it sounds tough, but I'm advocating doing this ALWAYS. Every day.

I'm telling you that if you want to achieve your best self and see a new you every day, then start eating ONLY when you have recently worked out.

Now, you've got three hours to eat, but it's OK to wait up to about one hour if you're not feeling hungry, but not more than two hours. To give you an example, here's my usual schedule for starting a great day (I am a bit of a morning person):

Patrick's Morning
8:00 am: Wake up. Feel grumpy.
8:30 am: Grab my coffee. Stop feeling grumpy.
9:00 am: Get to the gym and start my workout.
10:00 am: Wrap it up in the gym, end workout.
11:00 am: Start eating.
2:00 pm: Finish eating.

And by two in the afternoon, I'm done eating. After that, I don't eat for the rest of the day.

I was a two-hundred-pound (or so) male when beginning this diet, so I needed to eat about 2,300 calories a day (based on 12 calories/pound of goal weight per day and a goal weight of 190 pounds) and about 200 grams of protein (based on 1 gram per pound of goal body weight, rounded up from 190 grams). These amounts enabled me to lose body fat, not be miserable, and still have enough energy to work out.

Table 1. My stats

Month	Weight (lbs.)	Body fat %	Fat (lbs.)	Not fat (lbs.)
May	211	18	40	171
July	190	9	17	173

I lost a total of twenty-one pounds in seventy days. My body fat went down from 18 to 9 percent. I lost twenty-three pounds of fat and gained two pounds of muscle. I was ecstatic with my results, given that I didn't feel like I was actually working any harder. I was working smarter. I had just started using The NEW Ancient Diet for the first time officially—identical to the system it is today. And, it was easy, and just like that, I was ready for the beach.

So I apply fasting and my three-hour eating window, and every day I eat all of my 2,300 calories in the three hours between eleven in the morning and two in the afternoon, right after my daily workout.

This is custom-tailored to *my* needs and goals, and you might find different styles work better for you. If you're an evening person, then maybe you'll find it best to work out around five or six and then hit the fridge after that. Some people prefer to eat twice daily, and that's OK too; just divide your daily calories between the two meals, and make sure you work out before both of them.

It's also not a problem to play around with your workout and meal times to match your scheduling needs. For example, Sundays are pretty much free for me, so I sleep in, work out at a later time, and then eat at later time. Just remember that three hours is your magic number, and then let the system work for you.

Eating this way and training in a fasted state can help cure you of all symptoms of insulin resistance (you may be experiencing these symptoms whether or not you have been diagnosable with insulin resistance).

When you think about my method, it only makes more and more sense. Farmers, manual laborers, apex predators, kids, and athletes can eat tons of calories and not get tired or fat. They are very insulin-sensitive people. They are also people who, not coincidentally, often find them selves eating immediately after physical activity. All of these groups of people do tend to burn more calories than a sedentary adult, but they also freely consume more than enough food to make up for that.

There are many adults who are just as physically active as these groups but don't have the fitness level they wish they did. They exercise regularly and figure that if they're *consciously trying* to burn calories, then they should have the same metabolism as these groups that, albeit accidentally, apply proper caloric intake timing.

I sincerely hate to see it, because great people actually *work hard* at their fitness but aren't quite getting the results they want. If I could just get my ideas across to them, they could be achieving the higher levels of fitness they want *and deserve* with the same amount of effort *or even less.*

It's an old cliché, but its message runs thick in the veins of this book: you have to *work smarter, not harder.*

For a great example of proper caloric-intake timing, I say look no further than my four-year-old, Ivan. Almost every day, he's working and exercising hard out on the playground. As soon as he's done, he eats—*a lot.*

It might be more accurate for me to say that he inhales whatever you give him. Whether it's a peanut butter and jelly sandwich or an ice-cream sandwich, he'll keep eating them for as long as they keep coming.

With all that, he's still a fit kid. He's not overweight, and he certainly doesn't have any lack of energy. He sleeps well at night, dreaming softly of the playground, and the next day, he's right back on it.

It's easy to say that his metabolism is fantastic *because* he's a kid, and that's partly true, but unfortunately, childhood-obesity rates show that kids can put on weight just as adults do. Kids like Ivan, however, are great examples of maximum insulin sensitivity. Their lifestyle and eating habits are the way that they're meant to be, as mammals.

All of the apex predators of the wild (like Ivan, obviously) are unconsciously exercising perfect caloric-intake timing. Take a look at the bodies of lions, tigers, and wolves living in nature; they are lean and mean. Every single meal they have is first hunted, chased, and finally caught. There is no meal without physical activity first. Our species is meant to work for our food as well. Hunting and gathering and, later, farming or other manual labor have always been our norm.

The bottom line is that it's the nature of us humans, as mammals, to consume our food only after physical activity.

Farmers, apex predators, and Ivan the four-year-old all have never *actually thought about* timing their meals after exertion, but yet they all enjoy the benefits. There's no reason you can't have the same great health that comes with the optimal insulin sensitivity of a lion—you just have to *get to* the same optimal insulin sensitivity of a lion.

That's what I'm trying to teach you how to do. And the way to do it is by eating portions that are right for you *only after exercise* and daily fasting.

Some other Benefits of Fasting, Fasted Training and Caloric Intake Timing:

- ☺ Preferentially burn stored fat

- ☺ Improved glycogen storage capacity

- ☺ Increased anabolism and growth hormone, and decreased cortisol

- ☺ Improved body composition

- ☺ Resistance to fatness

GETTING STARTED

Getting into any new diet or exercise program can be intimidating, but starting The NEW Ancient Diet is simple once you make it work for you. The first several days may be a challenge. Get through those, and it gets much, much easier. In fact, it gets enjoyable.

A good example/recommendation for day one:

8:00 a.m.: Wake up.
8:30 a.m.: Drink a lot of coffee (or any non-caloric caffeinated beverage).
9:30 a.m.: Start workout.
10:30 a.m.: End workout.
11:30 a.m.: Start eating.
2:30 a.m.: Stop eating.

Enjoy the rest of your day.

To make the transition easier, I recommend applying only caloric-intake *timing* for the first three weeks, but not specific calorie control. That is, eat as much as you want for the first three weeks. Then apply timing AND specific calorie control after the first three weeks. Table 2 depicts this in detail.

Table 2. Long-term recommendations

Time	Food amount	Protein amount
First three weeks (fix insulin resistance)	As much as you want within about three hours after you work out	One gram per pound of goal body weight
After the first three weeks (lose max body fat)	Twelve calories per pound of goal body weight	One gram per pound of goal body weight

The time-line breakdown should look like this:

For the **first three weeks**, eat as much as you normally do, focusing on only doing so within your three-hour post-workout window.

After three weeks, still only eat within your three-hour window, but stick to your limit of twelve calories per pound of goal body weight per day. Protein is always one gram per pound of goal body weight.

Note that as long as you are making steady progress toward your goal (refer to chapter 5 for goal info), the system is working great. Keep up the good work.

PART TWO
THE GAME PLAN

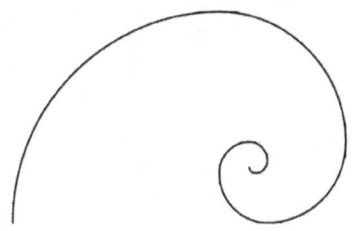

CHAPTER 4

THE FIRST THREE WEEKS

Everything should be made as simple as possible, but not one bit simpler.

—Albert Einstein

Now that you know the two key points to my method, you've already been handed the two most important tools I can give you. If you already have a workout regime that satisfies you, then the simple addition of those two steps *will* yield some great results. A lot of people will leave my book at this point, take the knowledge they have, and be better for it.

But for those of you who seriously want to take it to the NEXT LEVEL, this section's for you.

I'm going to introduce you to some great workouts tailor-made to complement my system to give you optimal results. First we focus on getting your insulin sensitivity back to the levels that will serve you best, and THEN we work on overhauling your body composition to get you looking perfect. All of my workouts seriously get your heart pumping and are going to get you to your absolute best.

Like I said, some of you may have a system that you're happy with and may not be looking for more information in this area. These workouts are for people who are looking to get 100-percent results from my system. Whether you don't have a regular workout routine yet or are looking for something new to push yourself to the next level, I got the 4-1-1 for you.

Fixing Insulin Resistance

The first step in finding your healthy *new* you is to get your insulin sensitivity back in check. If you're not obese and haven't noticed any of the major symptoms of insulin resistance, then you probably don't have a diagnosable condition, but you will still see major benefits when concentrating on getting yourself to the healthiest insulin sensitivity. In combination with proper eating, timing your calories, and fasting, use the workouts in this section to accomplish that (table 2, again, as a reminder).

Table 2. Long-term recommendations

Time	Food amount	Protein amount
First three weeks (fix insulin resistance)	As much as you want within three hours after you work out	One gram per pound of goal body weight
After the first three weeks (lose max body fat)	Twelve calories per pound of goal body weight	One gram per pound of goal body weight

The workouts in this section of The NEW Ancient Diet will challenge you; that's what they're meant to do. If you're having a tough time initially, it's OK to take it slow and progress to the full workout. As you get stronger, it will get easier, but you must always remember to *push yourself.* If a particular workout is easy enough that you can coast through it without too much effort, you're probably doing it wrong or going too light on the weights. It's OK if you have to push yourself.

Imagine a scale from one to ten that measures how much you're challenging yourself. We want these workouts to be between eight and ten. Remember that a level-eight-intensity workout isn't the same for everyone; a professional athlete or elite-level cross-fitter wouldn't even consider most of our tens to be a six on his scale. *And, that is OK.* Again, I want you to make sure that you are pushing *yourself.*

This isn't slow, restful cardio (see the FAQs section for further explanation); make sure your energy level is high and that each workout *is* a challenge. In other words, walking is not an acceptable exercise. Some people might argue that walking can be considered exercise. I am not one of those people. Walking (or any low-intensity activity) is not nearly intense enough to elicit the hormonal, fat loss, and insulin-sensitivity benefits that we want.

To challenge your self the most, I prefer heavy-resistance workouts (with weights) with short rest intervals. Workouts should last between thirty and ninety minutes, but *never* sacrifice intensity for duration. If thirty minutes becomes your normal workout length because of level of difficulty, *that's a good thing.*

> **Never, ever** sacrifice intensity for duration
>
> (It's in a box, so it must be important)

Women and men should generally be doing the same workout (again, see the FAQs section). Also, I have my criteria for a great workout that gets me pumped, but whatever workout you choose, make sure it follows some general rules:

- @ All major skeletal muscle groups should be activated throughout the week.

- @ You should definitely be breaking a sweat.

- @ A good gauge of intensity is whether or not you're able to speak. Your breathing should be heavy enough so that it's difficult for you to hold up any conversation past a quick, "Hey."

- @ Use ten to fifteen repetitions (reps), six sets (how many times you do the reps), and one-minute rest intervals between sets.

This rep and set scheme is ideal for improving insulin resistance, boosting the metabolism, encouraging fat loss, and maintaining muscle/strength.

- @ The ten to fifteen reps, six sets, and one-minute rest interval (wear a watch) needs to be challenging for you—an eight to ten intensity level. In other words, it *has gotta* be hard training with challenging weights.

@ Make sure to periodically increase the resistance (weight) or repetitions, because your body will adapt and get stronger as you get in shape. If you do it right, the same amount of weight soon won't be challenging enough. If you think it's getting too easy, it probably is. When in doubt, go heavy.

@ Remember the book of Genesis: get your body moving six days a week, but rest at least one.

The general workout that I designed and recommend for use with my system is this:

Day 1: lower body
Day 2: upper body
Day 3: athletic day—cardio and core
Day 4: lower body
Day 5: upper body
Day 6: athletic day—cardio and core
Day 7: rest
Day 8 and on: *rinse and repeat*

Now, by far the most important exercises you can do are those that activate multiple large muscle groups. Specifically and most importantly, activate the muscle groups behind you. That group of muscles has a name, "posterior chain," and because of its lack of immediate aesthetic appeal, it often gets secondary treatment to the glamour front muscles, or the chest and biceps.

The back, butt, thighs, hamstrings, and calves compose the posterior chain (thighs, although not part of the posterior chain, are also typically activated with posterior-chain exercises). Activating these groups is very important because it best recruits the most muscle possible, thus stimulating your metabolism maximally and burning the most body fat.

Activating the posterior chain bestows another benefit: it turns your butt into a *nice ass*! The kind that songs are written about.

> *My fantastic ass was built on bicep curls with pastel weights!*
>
> —No one

In descending order of greatness, remember these three posterior-chain exercises:

1. Barbell back squats: You get the most metabolism boost, the most muscle activated, and consequentially the most fat lost with the barbell back squat. Accept no substitutes. Did someone say, *she squats, bro!*

2. Barbell dead lifts: This is very similar to the squat, but the barbell dead lift places more emphasis on hamstrings and butt.

3. The Prowler: There is no better conditioning exercise. Enough said. Tell your gym manager to go to elitefts.com to buy one for the gym. It's worth the money.

You'll quickly realize that these are the three most challenging exercises in my system. But the fitness gods are just, and these workouts do reap the most rewards. Because they activate the posterior chain fully, these three exercises boast, by far, the most metabolism-boosting potential. Use these bad boys to help shape your body (and your backside) faster and to a greater extent than almost any other exercises. Make these three exercises the staples of your weekly workouts.

Note that what I'm saying is: *don't you dare skip leg day*. Leg days are sacred days when you must sacrifice to the workout gods to achieve levels of fitness mortals were never meant to know.

Another Note: You must get a gym membership. This is compulsory. The reason I really must insist on this is because most home gyms don't have the equipment you need, but most commercial gyms do. If finances are a concern, many areas have decent quality gyms for around ten to twenty bucks a month. Look on *Yelp*, try to find one that sounds like it's right for you, and then go check it out.

For a more specific example of an excellent comprehensive workout schedule, let's check out my friend Pam's typical workout:

Day 1 (lower body):

- Prowler (2 plates x 40 yards x 6 sets) with a two-minute rest interval

- ten-minute break

@ barbell back squats (115 pounds x 13 repetitions x 6 sets) with a two-minute rest interval

@ five-minute break

@ dumbbell walking lunges (40 pounds [20 pounds in each hand] x 21 repetitions x 6 sets) with a one-minute rest interval

Day 2 (upper body):

@ dumbbell shoulder press (25 pounds x 9 repetitions x 6 sets) with a one-minute rest interval

@ dumbbell chest press (35 pounds x 9 repetitions x 6 sets) with a one-minute rest interval

@ lat pull downs (90 pounds x 9 repetitions x 6 sets) with a one-minute rest interval

Day 3 (athletic day—cardio and core):

@ suicides on the basketball court (6 sets) with a one-minute rest interval

@ two-minute break

@ toe touches (while lying on your back, toes above you x as many as possible x 6 sets) with a thirty-second rest interval

@ barbell power cleans (85 pounds x 6 repetitions x 6 sets) with a one-minute rest interval

Day 4: repeat day 1 (except, substitute barbell deadlifts for barbell squats)

Day 5: repeat day 2

Day 6: repeat day 3

Day 7: off/cheat day

Let's go back to the main diet idea for this chapter.

To reiterate, you're trying to reset your insulin sensitivity to where it is *supposed to be* in a healthy, natural way. To accomplish this, you are to eat *only* within the three-hour (you can wait up to one hour) window after working out hard.

For the first 3 weeks, eat as much as you want:

Pizza?
Sure!

Wings and beer?
Go for it!

Chocolate?
Eat as much as you want!

Dry chicken breasts and rubbery broccoli?
Go for it! But you're kind of weird.

Other people?
No. Under no circumstance should you eat other people. Too caloric.

Eat whatever (just not whomever) and however much you want during this grace period, there are no limits.

But there is one minimum: strive daily to eat one gram of protein per pound of your goal body weight. This is a little on the high side, but it will help a lot to get used to this amount before your calories are lowered. It will also help satiate you, and it's *kind of incredibly important* for good body-composition management.

If your diet does not include adequate protein, remember that lean meats, fish, and eggs whites are all great sources. You may also consider investing in protein shakes. Many people (me included) love protein shakes because they load you up with whey protein and actually taste kind of freaking great.

Also remember that it's important to stay hydrated the rest of the day. Beyond your three-hour widow(s), you can have any non-calorie drinks: black coffee, diet soda, unsweetened tea, etc. And, of course, the drink of the fitness gods themselves: *water.* Avoid any beverages containing calories.

*Look, I eat really well and work out, but I also indulge
when I want to. I don't starve myself in an extremist way.
You're not taking away my dairy or my coffee or my wine,
because I'd be devastated.*

—Jennifer Aniston

Not the person you were expecting to be quoted in a diet book? Well
it's hard to disagree that Jen *still* has a heck of a bod, so whether it
seems like she's an authority on fitness or not, she kind of is.

And when she says that it's not necessary to entirely deprive yourself,
listen to her. This is what my book is *all about*. When you handle your
eating habits the way we humans, as mammals, were meant to, you'll
be surprised by just how little you have to sacrifice to enjoy the fitness
levels that you *deserve*. It **is** all about *timing* your calories and cutting
back a little. It *is not* all about restricting or eliminating the type of
food that you want and enjoy eating.

CHAPTER 5

DIALING IN

OK, you've completed your first three weeks of eating whatever you want but only after workouts (or you skipped ahead, I'm proud of you, overachiever), so what's next? Now that you have improved your insulin sensitivity greatly and lost some body fat, you are now ready to start working on decreasing your body fat to an even greater degree.

The best way to do that is to switch to eating fewer daily calories while still eating enough protein. This combo, fewer calories and enough protein, IS PROVEN to be ideal to shed maximum body fat, along with proper meal timing.

I want you to be strict with yourself about your daily calorie limits. Keep doing the workouts intensely to continue to keep your active muscle and hormones high, but start eating fewer calories.

Specifically, use twelve calories per pound of goal weight per day (calories/pound/day) as your limit. For example, if you want to be 150 pounds, then eat 1,800 calories a day and 150 grams of protein. That's your limit. It's not as hard as it seems, and once you've gotten used to the three-hour window, you'll be surprised at how little this feels like a sacrifice.

If you really, *really* don't want to go get your calculator, then check out the chart below to see how many calories and how much protein you should be eating daily.

Table 3. Daily calorie and protein amounts based on goal weight

Goal weight	Daily calories and protein
100 pounds	1,200 calories and 100 grams of protein
110 pounds	1,320 calories and 110 grams of protein
120 pounds	1,440 calories and 120 grams of protein
130 pounds	1,560 calories and 130 grams of protein
140 pounds	1,680 calories and 140 grams of protein
150 pounds	1,800 calories and 150 grams of protein
160 pounds	1,920 calories and 160 grams of protein
170 pounds	2,040 calories and 170 grams of protein
180 pounds	2,160 calories and 180 grams of protein
190 pounds	2,280 calories and 190 grams of protein
200 pounds	2,400 calories and 200 grams of protein
210 pounds	2,520 calories and 210 grams of protein
220 pounds	2,640 calories and 220 grams of protein

230 pounds	2,760 calories and 230 grams of protein
240 pounds	2,880 calories and 240 grams of protein
250 pounds	3,000 calories and 250 grams of protein
260 pounds	3,120 calories and 260 grams of protein
270 pounds	3,240 calories and 270 grams of protein
280 pounds	3,360 calories and 280 grams of protein
290 pounds	3,480 calories and 290 grams of protein
300 pounds	3,600 calories and 300 grams of protein
310 pounds	3,720 calories and 310 grams of protein
320 pounds	3,840 calories and 320 grams of protein
330 pounds	3,960 calories and 330 grams of protein
340 pounds	4,080 calories and 340 grams of protein

As far as protein intake goes, you'll notice that nothing has changed. I still want you eating one gram of protein per pound of goal body weight. If you want to weigh 150 pounds, that's 150 grams a day.

I know it's not what many of you want to hear, but your new fit lifestyle is going to have to involve the habit of reading nutritional-fact labels and weighing and measuring food. Don't let yourself be intimidated, it's actually pretty easy once you get the hang of it. I also suggest picking up a calorie info book like *Calorie King*. They can be great references for nutrition info on meats, fruits, veggies, restaurant fare, and even fast food.

Two important aspects of protein:

1. It is important to stress that you need to plan on the amount of protein to eat. So consider your amount of protein (think of lean meats, fish, and protein powder) for the day, and then add the rest of your calories to get to your limit. Since this is a higher protein diet, you will find that it is much easier when you make protein a priority.

2. Since protein is by far the most satiating food, it's a good idea to eat it last, toward the end of your meal and your three-hour window.

To recap, regarding protein: plan first, and eat last.

Here are some examples of 1,800 calories with 150 grams of protein.

1. Caesar salad with chicken, steak (twelve ounces raw weight), and three scoops protein powder

2. grilled shrimp salad, one slice cheesecake, and four scoops protein powder

3. two steak soft tacos, steak fajita meat (twelve ounces raw) with green and red veggies, and two large protein pancakes.

4. two cups pasta, one cup pasta sauce, six tablespoonfuls parmesan cheese, and two, eight-ounce chicken breasts

5. egg-white omelet (one cup egg whites from four large eggs, four cheese slices, and green and red veggies), one cup fried potatoes, and eight ounces yogurt

6. cod (twelve ounces raw), two cups fried rice, and a large spring roll with dipping sauce

ON MEASURING PROGRESS

You will need to measure your progress periodically while following The NEW Ancient Diet. This will ensure that you are on track to reach your goal.

It's possible to gauge your progress in many ways: body-composition changes, weight changes, how your clothes fit, inches lost, etc. To be as objective as possible, I would stick to only two: body-composition and body-weight changes.

How your clothes fit and inches lost are important, and some will prefer these rough measurements, but just like gauging how you feel, these can be hard to quantify. Because of this reason, I generally use weight and body composition changes to measure changes in body fat, only.

For weight changes, just buy an inexpensive bathroom scale, and you are ready to go. Or use the scale at the gym. Either one is OK, just *always* use the same scale. Also, the absolute accuracy of the scale is not that important; having that number go down over time is very important.

For body composition changes: measure your body fat using a device, such as calipers, bioelectrical impedance, underwater weighing or DEXA. Underwater weighing and DEXA are the most accurate methods. If those Cadillac versions aren't available to you, that's not a problem. *Any* method will work. More than likely, your gym will have either calipers or bioelectrical impedance. Either one is OK, just make sure that the operator is very familiar with the use of the device and that it's use is consistent every time you get measured.

Just get in the habit of checking your progress. I advise measuring your weight and body composition on a schedule. For example, do your measurements the morning of your weekly cheat day (for more on cheat days, read on).

Keep in mind that we are shooting for steady and measurable progress. Don't become obsessive. Measuring once or twice a week is fine.

EXPECTATIONS

Having said that, expect to lose one to three pounds (mostly fat) per week. Anything within that range is a normal and effective amount of weight loss.

I know what some of you are thinking: "I'll just cut calories even more than twelve per pound of goal weight per day!"

Well, I mean, you can absolutely do that, BUT if you cut calories too much more, there is *not* a guarantee that you will lose weight quicker. You do, however, guarantee that you'll be miserable. And being miserable makes it more likely that you'll quit dieting all together. The goal here is steady, measurable progress. Keep fighting my friend.

YOUR GOAL LINE

This is your chance to write down your goal while starting the NEW Ancient Diet. Keep in mind that your goal should be realistically attainable and measurable.

Write your goal here:

_____

Examples:

- @ lose fourteen pounds, starting May 1, by July 1

- @ get my body fat from 20 percent to 10 percent in three months, starting January 1

- @ go from 211 to 192 pounds in seventy days (This was my personal goal.)

PART THREE
A FINAL WORD

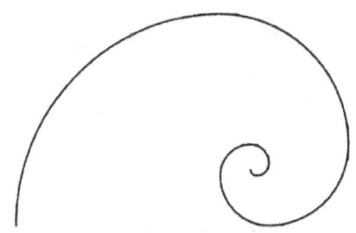

CHAPTER 6
NOTHING CAN STOP ME NOW

Above all, do not forget your duty to love yourself.
—Kierkegaard

I love myself, and I love who I am. I'm not afraid to say it. Sometimes our culture can make it seem like loving who you are is a bad thing, as if it is self-centered and narcissistic. But I say that loving who you are is actually self-accepting and optimistic. Are you, right now, able to say that you honestly love yourself and who you are?

It's an incredibly important question to ask yourself, and how you answer is maybe the single most crucial factor in determining how happy you are going to be in life. And, *yes,* your relationship *with yourself* is, without a doubt, the single most important relationship you will have in your life.

If you are lucky enough to be able to answer yes to this extremely important question, FANTASTIC. It is my hope that you are able to use this book to *earn the results* that will help you continue to celebrate YOU. Your happiness and self-value can only grow by using the tools I've given you.

If you can't say that you do love who you are, or if you're unsure how you would answer that question, then it's time to do something about it. It's time to improve your love of *yourself*. It's time to upgrade your self-worth and your self-esteem.

Your sense of self-worth is often tied in to your accomplishments. You *do* feel better about yourself when you have accomplished difficult things that are important to you. The fact that you're reading my book indicates that physical health is something that is important to you, and it *is* absolutely something worth earning. Because self-esteem also is often improved as you *work* and *better* your literal, physical self-image, once you change your body composition and shed body fat, your confidence will *soar*.

Testimonials about the fun side of dramatic weight loss almost always include increased energy and happiness once a person has reached his or her goal. But there are hundreds of studies to prove that exercise, in and of itself, increases energy and happiness and decreases depression. This is independent of reaching your goals.

Also, training in the fasted state and fasting in general have innate mental benefits that are independent of reaching your goals:

- increased energy

- increased focus

- increased sense of purpose

- increased autonomy

© increased happiness

© increased stress control

These mental benefits occur because of good stress. Hormesis is a term that describes that kind of stress.

HORMESIS

We humans are remarkably adapted to survive most stresses, good and bad, that are applied to us. Some specific stresses can cause positive adaptations, while others do not.

Hormesis is a term to describe beneficial stress that challenges the brain and body. This good-stress stimulates the brain, which then becomes stronger and thoughts become clearer. Stress hormones, such as adrenalin and serotonin, influence brain chemistry to adapt because of good-stress applied to it. And as your brain exercises through this new challenge with new hormone amounts, you become happier.

Fasting is a proven and ideal way to cause these adaptations (hormesis) to occur. As long as the fast does not last so long as to begin to have detrimental effects, positive adaptations occur. Twenty one-hour daily fasts are ideal, in my opinion, for *regularly* achieving hormesis without too much difficulty. It's not too long, but still long enough: just right. Working out in a fasted state just improves this *hormesis* from fasting to a much greater extent.

In truth, many scholars of psychology, religious and spiritual groups agree that fasting (hormesis) is REQUIRED for maximum happiness and clear thoughts. Look no further than some of the major religions of the world: Christianity, Islam, Judaism, Hinduism and Buddhism. All religions mentioned have an aspect of fasting involved in their faiths (And, in case you care, in all those religious texts, there is no mention of eating 3-6 times a day!) It is believed, in these religions, that fasting is directly connected to spirituality: which makes you more closely connected to God. So, it is easy to see how important fasting can be to place the brain in an optimal position for higher levels of thought, happiness and personal satisfaction which would translate to increased spirituality.

Let me break it down for you: this program is designed to most effectively cut body fat, hopefully leading to increased personal satisfaction, increased self-esteem and happiness when your goals are reached. AND, coincidentally, it's one of the best ways to activate hormesis and train your brain to *just be happier, before your goals are achieved.* This occurs just by starting and continuing The NEW Ancient Diet.

Despite all those benefits, some people don't want to start or are confused about where to begin. Some people don't like or care to work out and keep a steady watch on their diets. I completely understand that, because we, as people, will always tend toward ease. I would also argue, however, that those people haven't been given the correct motivation with the correct diet and exercise plan. In fact, once someone has the correct physical fitness and diet plan that works *for them* and *with them*, their outlook and energy will quickly adapt to help them achieve their goals. And keep in mind that I'm not asking you to become something different. I'm asking you to *discover who you were meant to be in the first place.*

Obviously no one is saying that your physical appearance will change dramatically overnight. It will absolutely take some time and commitment to get your dream body. But what I am saying is that you *will* feel better almost immediately from treating your body right.

While the hardest steps in any diet and exercise program are always the first, it only gets easier. It has a snowball effect, every time you exert your willpower to make a positive choice for your body, it becomes easier to do so the next time. That's how you are going to develop the great habits of the healthy person that you are going to become: one step at a time.

Today is the day.

Take control of your world.
Begin The NEW Ancient Diet.

NOW.

My publicist told me to include an inspirational haiku or homily here in the last chapter. I told him to stop using strange words that I don't understand. I then cleaned the spaghetti off of four-year-old Ivan's face and told him to whip something up.

I liked what he came up with, so I decided to share his ideas on how to motivate you, my beautiful reader, to achieve everything you can, and everything you *deserve*, to achieve. The kid had some pretty wise stuff he wanted to impart to you:

> It's not just about looking attractive and desirable to others. It's about looking good to yourself. It's about looking in the mirror and letting yourself believe that you are attractive.

> Once that happens, not only will you enjoy higher confidence levels than ever before, you will find your willingness and ability to stick to this diet and exercise program are both much stronger as well.

> Once you demand yourself to change your conscious self-image, your subconscious image of yourself will follow. This is when true confidence begins to flow through your spiritual being. At this point, when your subconscious has been amended, you are on easy street.

> Your subconscious is the true driving force of motivation in your life. As the goals that you have disciplined into your conscious thought sew themselves into your subconscious, they will begin to take form in your dreams coming true.

> This is you on the real road to happiness.

Once your dreams become your literal dreams, you will have accomplished the goals that you had desired and deserved. You will achieve your genetic potential and have a much greater satisfaction with who you are.

All of this is within you.

And the tool is in your hands. I urge you to take the first steps of your journey today.

Wow. Out of the mouths of babes, huh? I was so impressed that I forgot to wipe the sauce off of his cheek before he asked me if he could have some more "b'sgetti." (He can't pronounce "spaghetti" yet; it's pretty adorable.)

I don't know about you, reader, but I think that was crazy inspiring. Little Ivan did a pretty fantastic job.

I guess if my simpler mind had to summarize his points for the rest of us, he's saying that now you have the tool—**The NEW Ancient Diet**.

And now you need only to adhere, persevere, and accomplish your goals.

But, motivation is not unlike brushing your teeth; you gotta do it *each and every day*. You gotta practice and preach motivation to yourself daily. So when you're feeling overwhelmed or that it's not worth pursuing any further, here's a short list of tips to use for extra motivation:

- © **Workout planning:** Make plans to exercise: pack your exercise clothes beforehand, and make gym time a priority without giving yourself the option to skip. Maybe find a workout buddy so that you'll have more motivation to not bail. Keep detailed notes of your diet and exercise routines (you can use the notes and logs sections of this book).

@ *You are gorgeous. Keep up the good work!*

@ **Meal planning:** Plan your meals twenty-four hours in advance. In my experience, unless you do a little planning regarding what and when you are going to eat, it's easier to fail and cheat. Let's do what is necessary to avoid that and PLAN.

@ *All you need to change FOR THE BETTER is in your hands. It's been there all along.*

@ **Motivational pictures/quotes:** Place a motivating picture of you, someone else, or anything that motivates you to achieve your goals in a place that you can see daily. Clip or print out quotes that really speak to you, and stick them around. For example, I have a picture of myself at my goal weight and form on vacation in Vegas with my sister stuck to my refrigerator. Do I want to dig for a spud *in the fridge,* or do I want to look like a stud *on the fridge?*

@ **Visual Imagery**: Use your motivating picture to help conjure an image of yourself (in your head) for when you get to your goal weight. This is called visual imagery. So, close your eyes and use your imagination to put the conscious thought of your new body into your head. Take time for a few moments per day to practice this visual imagery. For example, do this before you workout and before you go to bed at night.

@ *You are a strong, adept, and beautiful apex human. Your ancestors bore this into your DNA. Don't let them down; don't ever give up.*

@ **Goals:** It's important to have distinct goals to push toward. These goals should be measurable, reasonable, and specific. Don't choose a vague goal, like, "I want to lose a lot of weight by next summer." Depending on your situation, that may be reasonable, but it's neither measurable nor specific. A better goal would be: "I want to lose fifteen pounds by June 1, starting April 1." Pick a goal today, write it down at the end of chapter 5, and stick to it.

@ *I love myself TODAY, just the way I am. Tomorrow even more.*

@ **Cheating**: Even if it sounds counterintuitive: I actually advise allowing yourself a sort of cheat day once a week. On that day, do whatever you feel like with meal timing, amount of food, type of food, etc. It's important, mentally and hormonally, to cheat or treat yourself periodically. Once a week is my preference.

(Cheat on your diet sometimes. Not yourself. Or your boyfriend. Or your girlfriend. Or your taxes. I'm not saying cheating on those things is OK. I'm just saying that it's OK to eat ice cream sometimes.)

I strongly advise actually letting yourself have this cheat day. In my experience, people who don't allow themselves a cheat *day* end up taking a cheat *week* or *month*. In other words, it's OK to bend so that you don't break. So plan a weekly cheat day, and take it. Make it your reward for a great week of sticking to your diet.

As an extra reminder: The goal of The NEW Ancient Diet is to get your body fat low to achieve your best self. I mean to *WOW* levels (9 to 21 percent body fat).

Don't lose sight of that goal.

And...

THE BIG SIX

1. It's easy: work out, and then eat. Also, there is very limited meal planning involved.

2. Limited hunger: once you become accustomed to it, you have almost no hunger. Compared to diets where you simply *eat less,* you'll feel quite satisfied.

3. No food-choice restriction: you can eat whatever you want.

4. Fast results: you will start to notice body-composition and mind changes immediately.

5. Effectiveness: this diet is simply the most effective way to get from *A* to *B*. You want to lose the most body fat? The NEW Ancient Diet is ideal for you.

6. Happiness: as your metabolism improves, The NEW Ancient Diet makes you mentally *sharper*, and it leads to making you happier as well. It doesn't even feel like you are on a diet.

Try not. Do, or do not. There is no try.

—Yoda

A final, final word...

Body-fat loss is what we're using to market this book as a product, and it *is* the goal *on the surface*. But really, *the end goal*—what I *really* hope this book honestly gets you—is happiness. Truly, happiness is the goal of all self-improvement. We are only on this great blue rock for a short while, and to be happy in those moments is all we can ask for.

Different people seek out personal satisfaction and, in turn, happiness in a lot of different places: jobs, family, relationships, religion, and so on. *How do you define happiness?* For me, the best way to find happiness has always been a strong connection between the body and the mind. When the mind and the body become strongly aligned with one another, joy of the spirit will follow.

There are two ways of getting there: you can improve the mind and hope that the body follows, or you can trust the best science and history to improve to your goal body to improve your mind. As you can tell, I advocate the latter. Make a decision to improve toward your goal body, and your mind will push you to get there and become less burdened by an unhealthy lifestyle. So make the decision today, and begin the journey. It may start out tough, but it gets easier every day.

> *You can't build a reputation on what you are going to do.*
> —Henry Ford

START.

RIGHT.

NOW.

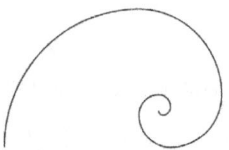

FAQs

@ **Do carbs make me fat?**

They can be the problem in some circumstances. It depends on a lot of variables, and it depends on your particular situation. I find that after correcting for protein intake, it doesn't matter all that much if you fill up the rest of your calories with fat, carbs, or any combo. Studies generally show this to be true, because when thinking about body composition, protein, calories, and timing, are the three most important aspects of your diet by a very wide margin.

Eat what you like and feels best for you, without violating calorie or protein limits. If it isn't working, then do some experiments with limiting carbs and/or fat, and stop when something works for you (That was the problem with the Atkins diet, a good idea for some but may not work best for others. Find what's right for you).

Having said that, generally carbs tend to be more appetite stimulating, so overeating can also be an issue. Keep that in mind.

⊚ Won't I get bulky from lifting weights?

If you're worrying about this, I assume you are one of my female read-ers. Well, to answer this question, you have nothing to worry about, and adding appropriate amounts of weight training to your program can only help. Unless you are using additional, um, supplements, the female body doesn't really produce the testosterone necessary to be-come very bulky. So generally, men get "swole" from weight training, and women get hot (not swole).

⊚ Will eating at night make me fat?

Nope. Total daily calories eaten against daily calories burned is, by far, the biggest determining factor in weight loss and gain. However, as far as stacking your calories at the beginning or the end of the day (breakfast versus late-night eating), hypo-calorie (under the amount that you need) studies have shown some differences, but the end result was that eating early in the day or later at night both produce similar weight-loss results.

For this reason, I advise just doing what appeals to you the most. If you like breakfast, eat breakfast. If you like eating late at night, then do that. You just have to have a workout completed first be-fore you eat. *#NeverForget*. (I'm just kidding. I'm not starting a damned hashtag.)

⊚ Isn't fasted cardio good for body-fat loss?

Short answer: kind of.

Long answer: as stated before, you *still* have to be in a negative calorie state to lose body fat. But regardless, I do highly encourage you to do your cardio fasted. It doesn't *directly* help your body lose extra fat to a great extent, but it does *indirectly* yield substantial benefits because of how much you'll be increasing your insulin sensitivity. In fact, I encourage you to do all your exercise in a fasted state (kind of a major part of this book).

Note: I prefer you do high-intensity (weight) training, etc., over steady-state cardio.

Now, I certainly don't want to alienate my cardio-o-phile readers by stating that. But my view is this: long, slow, boring, non-challenging cardio (steady-state) is not that beneficial.

The negatives:

@ When you do steady-state cardio, you aren't burning that many calories (one hundred to two hundred). That's just a lot of time and effort exerted for weaker results.

@ There aren't that many hormonal adaptations with steady-state cardio, compared to resistance training. Endorphins, dopamine, growth hormone, serotonin, adrenalin, testosterone, and so on all increase with intense exercise, but not so much with steady-state cardio.

@ When you do steady-state cardio, you don't get much after effect as far as calories burned. So when you stop the cardio, the calorie burning stops too. However, when you do resistance training, you burn a lot of calories *after the actual workout*—for up to twenty-four hours after the training session.

The positives:

© It is *certainly* better than not working out at all.

© It will improve your insulin sensitivity a bit more.

My recommendation for you cardiohards: if your cardio is *not* steady-state, that's when the real action happens.

We in the fitness business call it HIT (high-intensity training), or intervals or intermittent training, etc. You basically mix up the intensity of your workout (the opposite of *steady state*). For example, you train hard for a minute, rest a minute, train hard for a minute, rest a minute, and so on, for about thirty minutes.

I'm a fan of HIT. Time-wise, it's definitely one of the most efficient ways to burn and after-burn calories. In this sense, it's very similar to heavy-weight training for ten to fifteen repetitions. So I'm not necessarily against cardio—not at all. As long as the intensity is high enough, no matter what you do, you will reap enough rewards for the time you put in.

© **Can I drink alcohol while on this diet?**

Short answer: kind of. (Sorry to keep doing this to you.)

Long answer:

Alcohol is one of the most calorific substances on the planet.
—Ozzy Osbourne

Here's the bad news: you still have to fit all of your boozing into the calorie limits that you set for yourself. This will obviously be easier on cheat day, when you get to go off of the rails like a crazy train, but as you get into counting calories, you'll find that the Oz-man wasn't just being paranoid. He was laying down the hard truth. It's OK to have a drink while you're out with friends, but it can be pretty easy to let yourself have a few more and then watch your calorie limit flying high again. So when you find yourself thinking, "I don't wanna stop," maybe consider skipping the next round to hit the gym to pump some iron, man.

© **Doesn't eating six meals a day keep my metabolism higher?**

Short answer:

Noooooooooooooooo!
—Luke Skywalker

The difference between six small meals and one large meal has only a small effect on your metabolism, and if anything, one meal a day plays more to your favor. The composition of your meals (protein, fat, and carbohydrates) does matter, as does timing of your calories in relation to your workout. The idea of eating six meals a day to keep your metabolism high, however, is pure fallacy.

This idea comes from (often needled) bodybuilders, who really do need to eat 5,000-plus calories a day to keep their mass. They have to eat so much food, in fact, that it might be impractical for them to attempt to fit it all in at one meal (though they would still yield similar benefits if they did). Six meals a day does work well for *extreme bodybuilders*, but this method should have never found its way into mainstream dieting. For the average person on a normal or reduced-calorie diet, one meal a day is a healthier and more natural way to optimize your body composition.

Other negatives to eating six times a day:

- © A lot of meal planning is involved.

- © It can be difficult to follow. Your life suddenly is all about when you eat next.

- © Insulin is always high to medium high. That means hunger is always hanging around.

© **Isn't breakfast the most important meal of the day?**

> *Alas, my brethren, I speak true to thee: our father in heaven hath created all meals of the day equal, and thou shall not exalt breakfast before thine other meals.*
>
> —I made this up.

But I didn't make up the facts. Breakfast isn't special. In fact, eating arbitrarily when you *aren't even hungry*, just because you've been told it's good for you, is actually kind of a bad idea. People are told breakfast is important because of the presumption that it kicks your metabolism up for the rest of the day—and that's it's good for you. I'm actually here, with this book, to challenge that presumption. Just because it's the established norm doesn't mean that eating three meals a day is the healthiest way to live. Challenge the norm with me, and see the results for yourself.

℮ Won't I lose muscle if I train fasted?

Aha, trying to trick me now? The answer is no, this won't be a problem. Your body does need food and energy after training (within three hours, preferably), and you're still giving it what it needs. Problems with muscle loss might arise if you don't eat for longer than twenty-four to forty-eight hours, which you generally won't be doing and is not something I'm advocating as a part of my program (If you end up doing this for separate health or religious reasons, it still shouldn't mess things up too much). Otherwise, normal daily fasting does not lead to muscle loss.

℮ Should I be eating organic and natural food?

Organic food is not a necessary part of my program. Current regulations allow for loose definitions of the term "organic" to be used when marketing products, and I understand that the cost can be a burden for many.

There is little to no research to suggest that organic versus nonorganic food has any effect on *body composition*, which is the focus of my book and my diet. Organic is important to many people, and some will even have a small selection of products that they buy organic without their other groceries being organic. Both of these views are great, and while

I won't disparage them, I'm not advocating them as a necessary part of my dieting program.

@ **Will abdominal exercises get me a six-pack?**

This isn't a question people ask *me*, as much as it is a question that people ask *often*, and I wanted to clear some things up. Abdominal exercises can do a lot to strengthen the core (which is important for performance and to build muscle mass), but the myth of spot-fat reduction is a lie, a fakery, a two-horned unicorn.

A six-pack is all about your body fat percentage, which represents your *total* body fat throughout your entire body. You have to earn your abs my friend, by shedding the fat with meal timing and lower calories.

@ **How important is it to eat clean?**

"Eating clean" can be a pretty vague phrase. Everyone has his or her own idea of what this means. In general, if eating clean means consuming food that is natural and unprocessed, then, yes, it can be better for you in regard to different health markers. But again, my diet focuses on body composition, shedding fat, and maintaining muscle. With these goals in mind, I look at overall calorie intake and protein as the most important factors. Eating clean can be great for other health issues, but because of higher cost and lower taste, I take the same stance I have in regard to organic: it's not necessary here.

@ **A lot of people put heavy emphasis on drinking large amounts of water; how much water should I be drinking?**

Short answer: enough. (Aha! Cryptic.)

Long answer: With regulatory homeostatic hormones, the human body is uniquely adapted to survive during periods of more and less water availability. If you drink a little less water than normal, then your body retains more of it, and you urinate less out. If you drink too much water, your body will just urinate all the excess out. Obviously drinking extremely little water is bad, so do avoid that, and drink whenever you are thirsty. *Just a bit* more than you need to not get thirsty is about right. Any more than that doesn't yield additional benefits; you're just sending yourself to the bathroom more often.

That being said, many argue that drinking more water keeps you from drinking different, high-calorie drinks. If you are one of the people making this argument, then it probably does work for you. I won't tell you to go and make sure you drink two gallons of Arrowhead a day, but if you find that having a water bottle nearby helps you from ordering a sugary Coke, then by all means, drink up. Water is the nectar of the fitness gods.

(Gatorade will probably try to sue me for saying that.)

(Let them, Ivan's studying to take the bar exam in a month.)

ⓒ Should I limit my salt intake?

In the context of body composition, unless you are salt-sensitive, salt intake has little bearing. If you are salt-sensitive, then you may already struggle with high blood pressure, and you should talk to your doctor. If you're not salt-sensitive, then just keep everything *moderate* (don't dump the salt on your potatoes for ten seconds straight), and you should be fine.

℗ Is there a gender difference when considering exercise selection?

It's surprising to many, but not really. Both genders have the same muscle groups and cardiovascular system and, thus, will generally benefit from the same workouts in the same ways.

The only real difference is that the genders do seem to have different workout *preferences*. Men, more than women, are probably going to focus on working out their biceps to get nicer guns, and women are probably going to be more focused on working out their glutes to get nicer buns.

Whoa. Did that rhyme? Someone tell Sir Mix-a-Lot to hang up the pen or he's got himself a war.

℗ Isn't exercising enough? Do I really have to diet?

With fitness, doing anything is better than doing nothing, but every piece that you add makes it even better. If lower body fat and optimal body composition is your goal, then proper dieting is paramount. Both diet and exercise are very important, in tandem. Adding proper caloric-intake timing to exercise can help things—A LOT, even if you're not on a strict diet, but I always recommend proper dieting as well.

Remember: you can't out-train a bad diet.

@   **I have a really bad back, so I can't exercise. Isn't dieting enough?**

If you really do have a serious, diagnosed issue with your back, I'm sorry for that, and I recommend seeing a doctor. If you have a minor issue with your back, I still recommend seeing a doctor.

Exercise is vitally important to a healthy lifestyle. Don't let yourself become bedridden and watch your health decline because of a bad back. Find a way to make it work, and become who you deserve to be.

See the Health Checkup section, and consult a doctor if you have to. Some issues actually can get in the way of a proper exercise routine. Other issues end up being nothing more than crutches we allow ourselves so that we feel OK not pushing our limits to achieve our best...

@   [**Insert other** *excuses* **here**: a bad thyroid, bad metabolism, bad genetics, etc.]

Oh my goodness. I'm so sorry, I understand.

It's OK, I know. I know. Life is hard.

It's OK. Everyone understands. They get it.

It's OK. There's a reason you're not achieving your goals. And they understand.

They do understand [**excuse**].

But they're not going to fix it for you.

But [**excuse**] isn't going to turn them on. They're not going to find your excuses as attractive as the person *you're going to be* when you get out and make your goals your realities.

If you want an excuse not to do it, you'll find it.

But if you believe in yourself, others will begin to believe in you too.

The power to change your own life is currently in your hands.

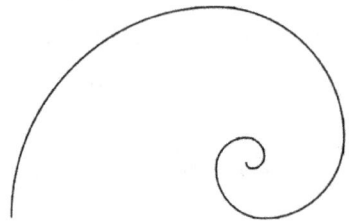

NOTES

DIET LOG

Exercise Log

HEALTH CHECKUP

If you're planning to increase your physical activity or start an exercise program, you should begin by answering a few questions. The PAR-Q (Physical Activity Readiness Questionnaire) is the gold standard in fitness safety. Doctors, trainers, and health clubs the world over use it. Usually comprised of five to seven questions, it can help rule out any underlying health concerns that could worsen with exercise. Answer yes or no to the following questions:

© Has your doctor ever said that you have a heart condition and that you should only do physical activity recommended by a doctor?

© Do you feel pain in your chest when you do physical activity?

© In the past month, have you had chest pain when you were not doing physical activity?

◎ Do you lose your balance because of dizziness, or do you ever lose consciousness?

◎ Do you have a bone or joint problem (for example, back, knee, or hip) that could be made worse by a change in your physical activity?

◎ Is your doctor currently prescribing drugs (for example, water pills) for your blood pressure or heart condition?

◎ Do you know of any other reason why you should not do physical activity?

If you answer YES to any of the questions on this list, you must check in with your doctor and get cleared for exercise before you start.

Likewise, if you have any chronic medical conditions (such as diabetes, high blood pressure, or arthritis) or risk factors (such as smoking or being more than twenty pounds overweight) and have not discussed exercising with your doctor, you should do so before beginning. Exercise is often an important part of the treatment for such conditions, but you may have some limitations or special needs that your doctor can tell you about.

ABOUT THE AUTHOR

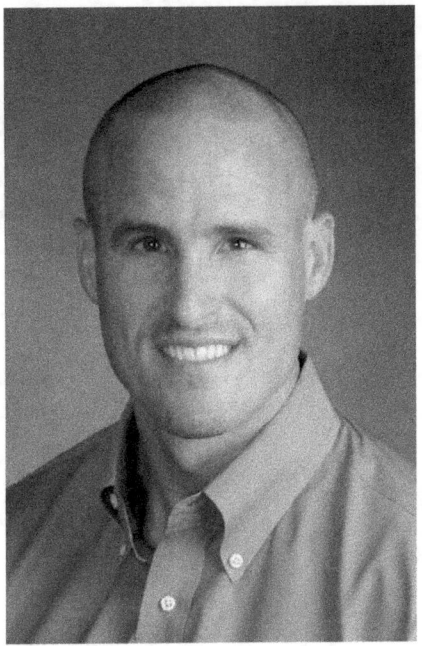

Patrick D. Espy, MS, RPh, is a practicing pharmacist, trainer, science nerd, and fitness expert. He graduated from Ohio State University with a bachelor's degree. Also, he has a master's degree in exercise physiology from Arizona State University, with emphasis on hormonal interactions with diet and exercise. For over twenty years, he has been working in the health care and fitness industry. His singular goal and dedication is in helping others to get lean, healthy, and feel and look amazing!

REFERENCES

M. Alirezaei et al., "Short-Term Fasting Induces Profound Neuronal Autophagy," *Autophagy* 6 (2010): 702–710.

R. M. Anson et al., "Intermittent Fasting Dissociates Beneficial Effects of Dietary Restriction on Glucose Metabolism and Neuronal Resistance to Injury From Calorie Intake," *Proceedings of the National Academy of Sciences of the United States of America* 100 (2003): 6216.

P. J. Arciero et al., "Increased Protein Intake and Meal Frequency Reduces Abdominal Fat During Energy Balance and Energy Deficit," *Obesity* 7 (2013): 1357–1366.

S. Awad et al., "The Effects of Fasting and Refeeding With a 'Metabolic Preconditioning' Drink on Substrate Reserves and Mononuclear Cell Mitochondrial Function," *Clinical Nutrition* (Edinburgh, Scotland) 29 (2010): 538–544.

B. Bahadori et al., "'Mini-Fast With Exercise' Protocol for Fat Loss," *Medical Hypotheses* 73 (2009): 619–622.

E. Bouhlel et al., "Ramadan Fasting Effect on Plasma Leptin, Adiponectin Concentrations, and Body Composition in Trained Young Men," *International Journal of Sports Metabolism* 18 (2008): 617–627.

U. Bradley et al., "Low-Fat Versus Low-Carbohydrate Weight Reduction Diets: Effects on Weight Loss, Insulin Resistance and Cardiovascular Risk, A Randomized Control Trial," *Diabetes* 58 (2009): 2741–2748.

A. J. Bruce-Keller et al., "Food Restriction Reduces Brain Damage and Improves Behavioral Outcome Following Excitotoxic and Metabolic Insults," *Annals of Neurology* 45 (1999): 8–15.

J. D. Cameron, M. J. Cyr, and E. Doucet, "Increased Meal Frequency Does Not Promote Greater Weight Loss in Subjects Who Were Pescribed an 8-Week Equi-Energetic Energy-Restricted Diet," *British Journal of Nutrition* 103, no. 8 (2010): 1098–1101.

O. Carlson et al., "Impact of Reduced Meal Frequency Without Caloric Restriction on Glucose Regulation in Healthy Normal-Weight Middle-Aged Men and Women," *Metabolism* 56 (2007): 1729–1734.

A. W. Chibalin et al., "Exercise-Induced Changes in Expression and Activity of Proteins Involved in Insulin Signal Transduction in Skeletal Muscle: Differential Effects on Insulin Receptor Substrates 1 and 2," *Proceedings of the National Academy of Science of the United States of America* 97 (2000): 38–43.

B. W. Craig, R. Brown, and J. Everhart, "Effects of Progressive Resistance Training on Growth Hormone and Testosterone Levels in

Young and Elderly Subjects," *Mechanisms of Ageing and Development* 49 (1989): 159–169.

K. De Bock et al., "Exercise in the Fasted State Facilitates Fibre Type-Specific Intramyocellular Er Lipid Breakdown and Stimulates Glycogen Resynthesis in Humans," *Journal of Physiology* 564 (2005): 649–660.

L. Deldicque et al., "Increased p70s6k Phosphorylation During Intake of Protein-Carbohydrate Drink Following Resistance Exercise in the Fasted State," *European Journal of Applied Physiology* 108 (2010): 791–800.

K. Fox, "The Influence of Physical Activity on Mental Well-Being," *Public Health Nutrition* 1999; 2: 411–418.

C. D. Gardner et al., "Comparison of the Atkins, Zone, Ornish, and LEARN Diets for Change in Weight and Related Risk Factors Among Overweight Premenopausal Women—The A to Z Weight Loss Study: A Randomized Clinical Trial," *Journal of the American Medical Association* 297 (2007): 969–977.

W. Duan and M. P. Mattson, "Dietary Restriction and 2-deoxy-glucose Administration Improve Behavioral Outcome and Reduce Degeneration of Dopaminergic Neurons in Models of Parkinson's Disease," *Journal of Neuroscience Research* 57 (1999): 195–206.

V. K. Halagappa et al., "Intermittent Fasting and Caloric Restriction Ameliorates Age-Related Behavior: Deficits in the Tripe-Transgenic Mouse Model of Alzheimer's Disease," *Neurobiology of Disease* 26 (2007): 212–220.

N. Halberg et al., "Effect of Intermittent Fasting and Refeeding on Insulin Action in Healthy Men," *Journal of Applied Physiology* 99 (2005): 2128–2136.

K. Y. Ho et al., "Fasting Enhances Growth Hormone Secretion and Amplifies the Complex Rhythms of Growth Hormone Secretion in Man," *Jounal of Clinical Investigation* 81 (1988): 968–975.

P. T. Jabekk et al., "Resistance Training In Overweight Women On a Ketogenic Diet Conserved Lean Body Mass While Reducing Body Fat," *Nutrition and Metabolism* (Lond) 7 (2010): 17.

D. Jakubowicz et al., "High Caloric Intake at Breakfast vs. Dinner Differentially Influences Weight Loss of Overweight and Obese Women," *Obesity* 21 (2013): 2504–2512.

C. S. Johnstone et al., "Ketogenic Low-Carbohydrate Diets Have No Metabolic Advantage Over Nonketogenic Low-Carbohydrate Diets," *American Journal of Clinical Nutrition* 83 (2006): 1055–1061.

W. J. Kraemer et al., "Endogenous Anabolic Hormonal and Growth Factor Responses to Heavy Resistance Exercise in Males and Females," *International Journal of Sports Medicine* 12 (1991): 228–235.

W. J. Kraemer et al., "Hormonal and Growth Factors to Heavy Resistance Exercise Protocols," *Journal of Applied Physiology* 69 (1990): 1442–1450.

G. N. Kraniou, D. Cameron-Smith, and M. Hargreaves, "Acute Exercise and GLUT4 Expression in Human Skeletal Muscle: Influence of Exercise Intensity," *Journal of Applied Physiology* 101 (2006): 934–937.

W. J. Kraemer et al., "Endogenous Anabolic Hormonal and Growth Factor Responses to Heavy Resistance Exercise in Males and Females," *International Journal of Sports Medicine* 12 (1991): 228–235.

G. N. Kraniou, D. Cameron-Smith, and M. Hargreaves, "Effect of Short-Term Training on GLUT-4 mRNA and Protein Expression in Human Skeletal Muscle," *Experimental Physiology* *89* (2004): 559–563.

A. E. Larsen et al., "Actions of Short-Term Fasting on Human Skeletal Muscle Myogenic and Atrogenic Gene Expression," *Annals of Nutrition and Metabolism* 50 (2006): 476–481.

J. Lee, J. P. Herman, and M. P. Mattson, "Dietary Restriction Selectively Decreases Glucocorticoid Receptor Expression in the Hippocampus and Cerebral Cortex of Rats," *Experimental Neurology* 166 (2000): 435–441.

P. Mansell, I. W. Fellows, and I. A. Macdonald, "Enhanced Thermogenic Response to Epinephrine After 48-h Starvation in Humans," *American Journal of Physiology* 258 (1990): R87–93.

M. P. Mattson and R. Wan, "Beneficial Effects of Intermittent Fasting and Caloric Restriction on the Cardiovascular and Cerebrovascular Systems," *Journal of Nutritional Biochemistry* 16 (2005):129–137.

M. P. Mattson, W. Duan, and Z. Guo, "Meal Size and Frequency Affect Neuronal Plasticity and Vulnerability to Disease: Cellular and Molecular Mechanisms," *Journal of Neurochemistry* 84 (2003): 417–431.

M. Noakes et al., "Comparison of Isocaloric Very Low Carbohydrate/ High Saturated Fat and High Carbohydrate/Low Saturated Fat Diets on Body Composition and Cardiovascular Risk," *Nutrition and Metabolism* (Lond) 3 (2006): 7.

I. Shai et al., "Weight Loss With a Low-Carbohydrate, Mediterranean, or Low-Fat Diet," *New England Journal of Medicine* 359 (2008): 229–241.

M. R. Soeters, "Intermittent Fasting Does Not Affect Whole-Body Glucose, Lipid, or Protein Metabolism," *American Journal of Clinical Nutrition* 90 (2009): 1244–1251.

S. Sofer et al., "Greater Weight Loss and Hormonal Changes After 6 Months Diet With Carbohydrates Eaten Mostly at Dinner," *Obesity* 19 (2011): 2006–2014.

S. R. Stannard et al., "Adaptations to Skeletal Muscle With Endurance Exercise Training in the Acutely Fed Versus Overnight-Fasted State," *Journal of Science and Medicine in Sport* 13 (2010): 465–469.

B. R. Stephens et al., "Effect of Timing of Energy and Carbohydrate Replacement on Post-Exercise Insulin Action," *Applied Physiology, Nutrition and Metabolism* 32 (2007): 1139–1147.

K. S. Stote et al., "A Controlled Trial of Reduced MKeal Frequency Without Caloric Restriction in Healthy, Normal-Weight, Middle-Aged Adults," *American Journal of Clinical Nutrition* 85 (2007): 981–988.

K. Van Proeyen et al., "Training in the Fasted State Improves Glucose Tolerance During Fat-Rich Diet," *Journal of Physiology* 588 (2010): 4289–4302.

K. A. Varady et al., "Improvements in Body Fat Distribution and Circulating Adiponectin by Alternate-Day Fasting Versus Calorie Restriction," *The Journal of Nutritional Biochemistry* 21 (2010):188–195.

K. A. Varady, "Intermittent Versus Daily Calorie Restriction: Which Diet Regimen is More Effective for Weight Loss?" *Obesity Rev* 7 (2011): 593–601.

J. F. Wojtaszewski et al., "Insulin Signaling and Insulin Sensitivity After Exercise in Human Skeletal Muscle," *Diabetes* 49 (2000): 325–331.

C. Zauner et al., "Resting Energy Expenditure in Short-Term Starvation is Increased as a Aesult of an Increase in Serum Norepinephrine," *American Journal of Clinical Nutrition* 71 (2000): 1511–1515.

H. Zhu, Q. Guo, and M. P. Mattson, "Dietary Restriction Protects Hippocampal Neurons Against the Death-Promoting Action of a Presenilin-1 Mutation," *Brain Research* 842, no. 1 (1999): 224–229.

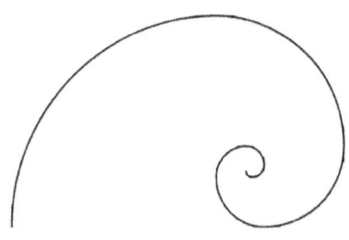